Dear Diary, I'm Going to a Birthday Party!

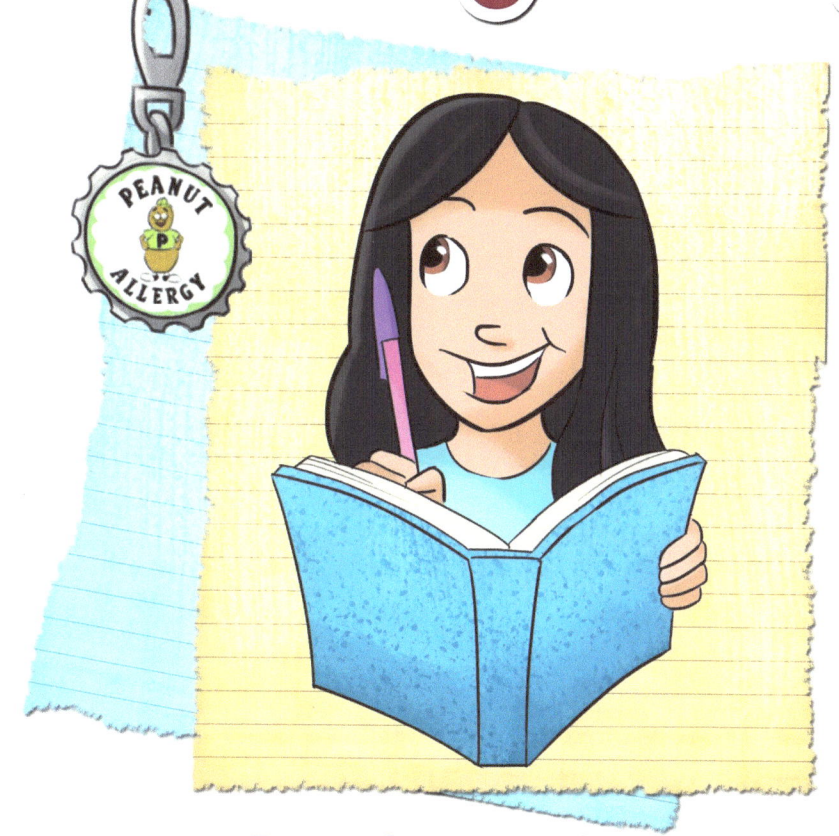

By Kathy Argel

Illustrated by Marvin Alonso

Dear Diary, I'm Going to a Birthday Party!

Copyright © 2017 by Kathy Argel

This book is dedicated to

Tristan & Nina

You are my inspirations.
Live your life to the fullest.
Have courage and be kind because
everyone has a story. I love you both
always.

Acknowledgement

Thank you to **Roland**, my husband, for supporting my dreams no matter how big or small. It's because of you I'm always reaching for the stars.

Visit **www.allergykidscentral.com** for more information.

"Always consult with a physician for the best food allergy plan and treatment for your unique situation."

This Book Belongs To:

Nina Packer

Certified Allergy Kid

ABOUT ME

Name: Nina Packer

FAV Colors: Green, blue, purple, pink, violet

FAV Snacks: Ice cream and cupcakes!

BFF's: Gracie, Gabby, Tori

School: Eagle Elementary School

FAV Things To Do: Create, draw, paint

(basically all artsy stuff!)

Allergies: Peanuts, tree nuts

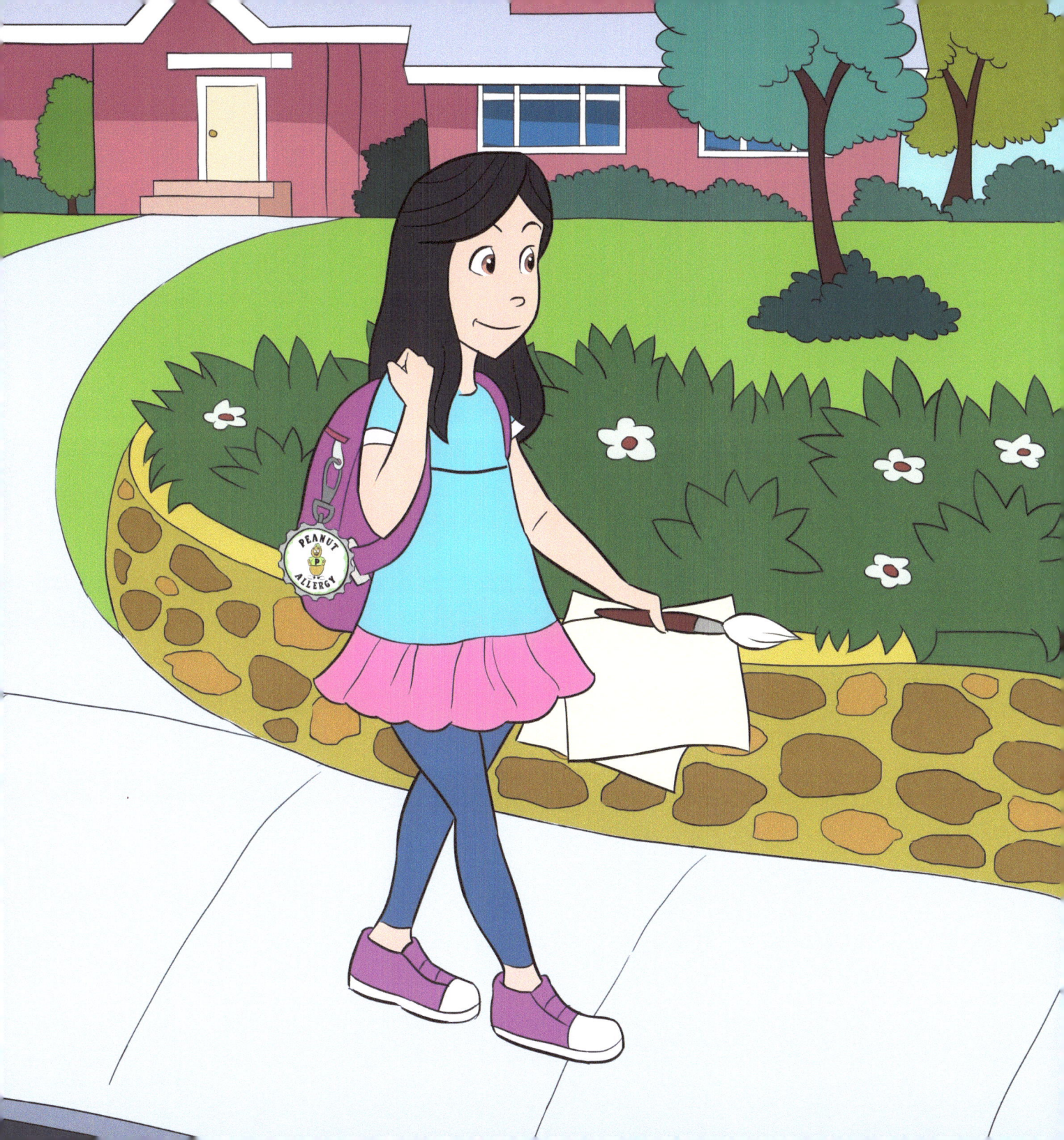

~ SATURDAY ~

Dear Diary,

I can't even tell you how I feel right now! I just got an invitation to Gracie's birthday party! I feel 87 % AWESOME, and 13 % NERVOUS. I feel awesome because the party is at Sport Zone, only the most awesome place ever! All my best friends are gonna be there! But I feel nervous because I have food allergies. I've been to parties before, but every party is different.

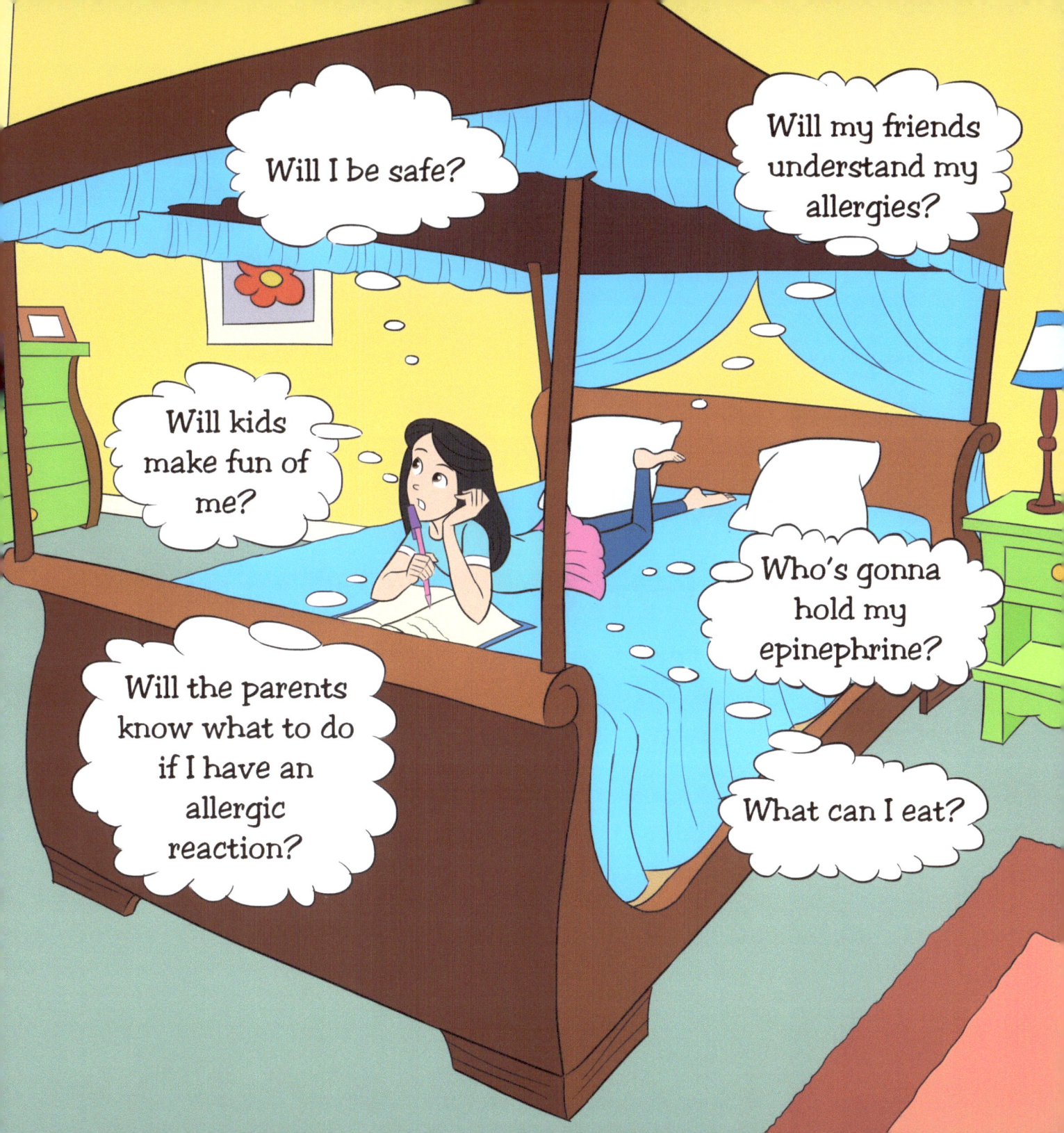

~SUNDAY~

Dear Diary,

I can't wait for the party! Six more days till the big event! I think I'll talk to my mom about my concerns. She's a great listener and loves me very much. Together, we'll make a plan!

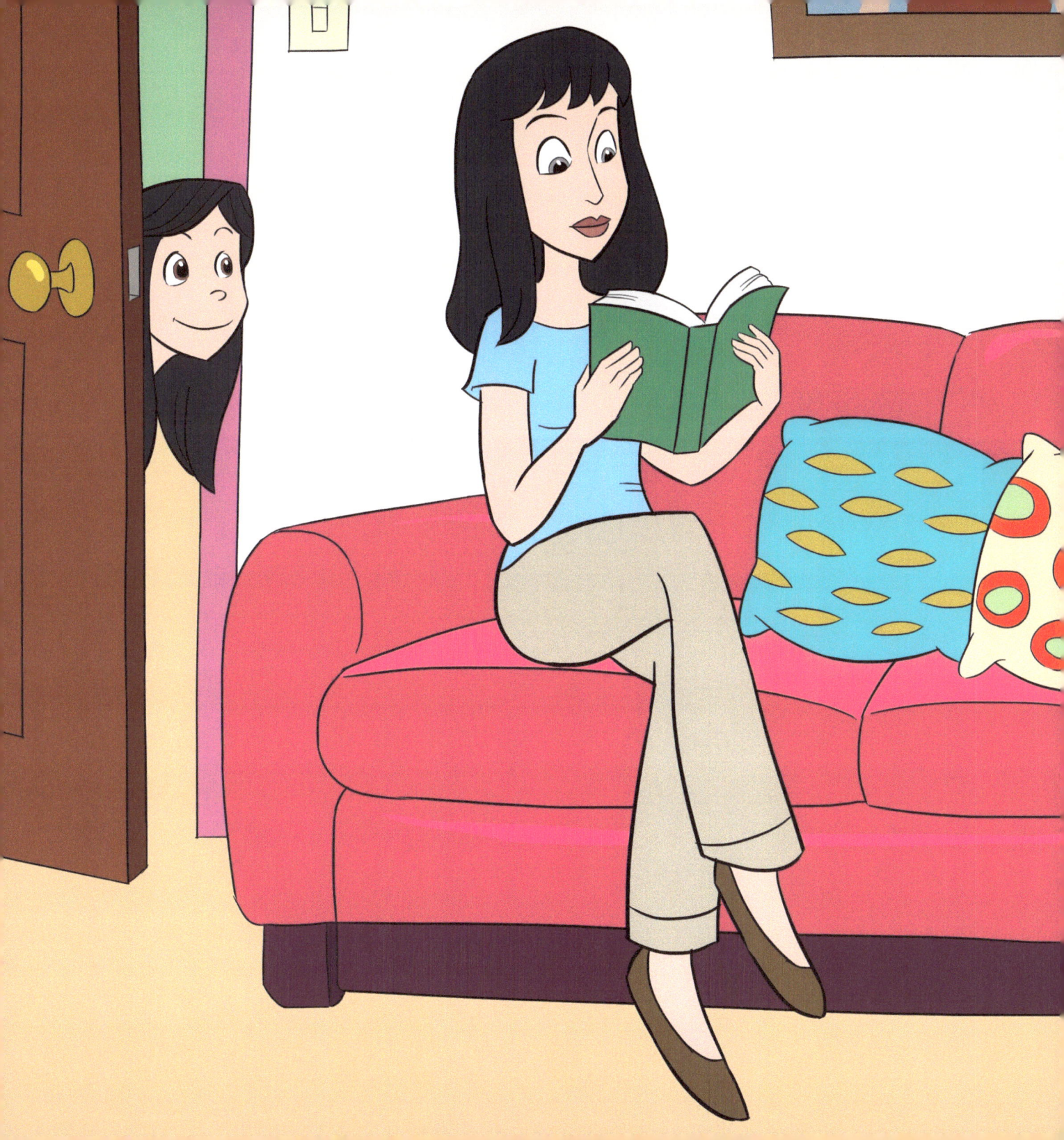

~ MONDAY ~

Dear Diary,

At school today, all my friends were talking about the birthday party. I'm so excited. Oh wait — I still need to RSVP for Gracie's party! I'm so excited! My mom and I still need to come up with a plan.

Will they have treats with nuts? Who can I talk to in case I get sick? Will I have fun if all I do is worry? I wish I didn't have to always worry about my food allergies. ☹

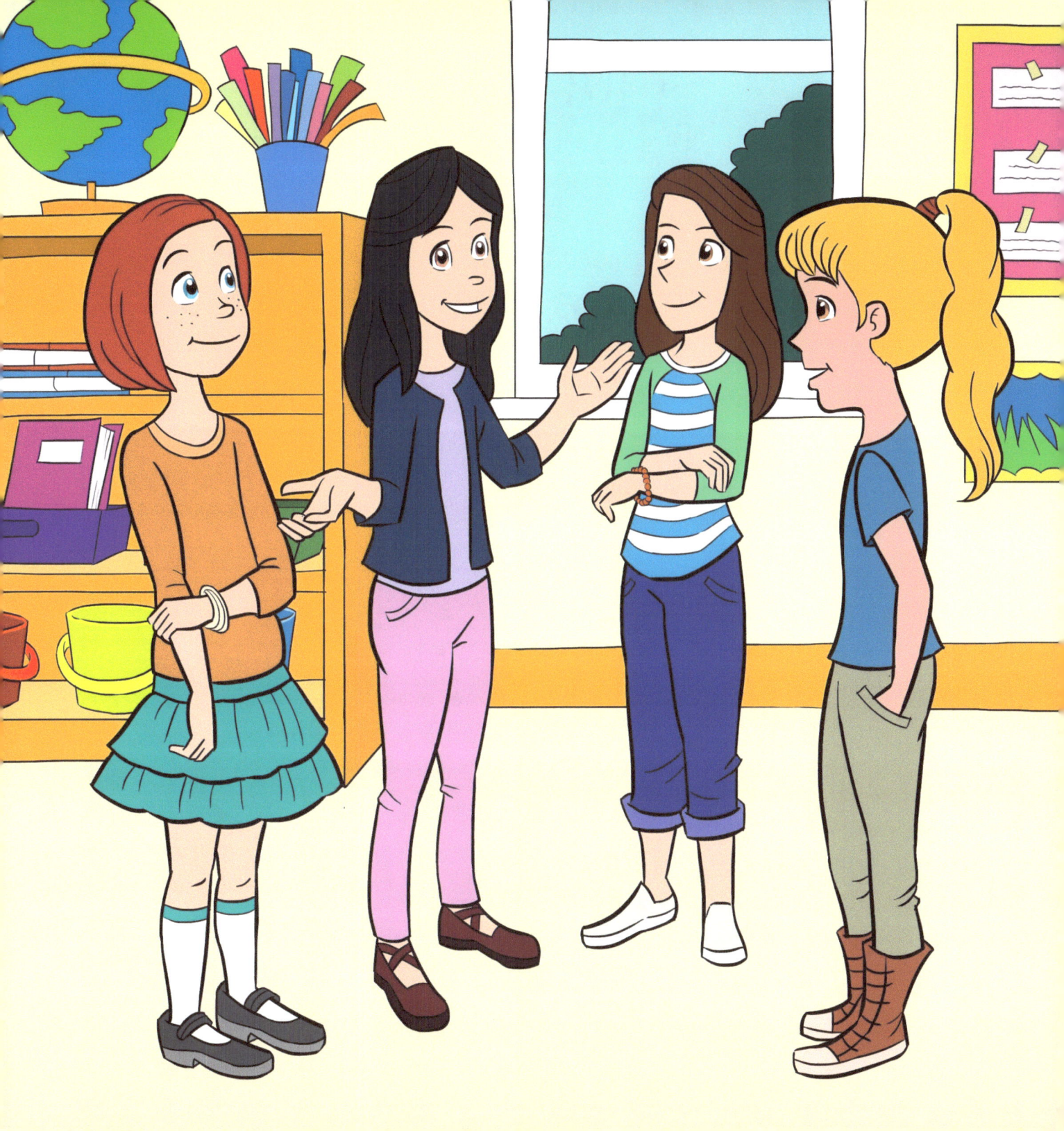

~ TUESDAY ~

My mom spoke with Gracie's mom about my food allergies. Together, we've come up with a plan!

My Plan

What food are they gonna serve?

PIZZA! Gracie's mom is getting it at my favorite restaurant, so I know it's safe! Gracie's mom ROCKS!

Desserts?

Cupcakes!
But, I can't have them because they might have nuts in them. Gracie's mom can't cook allergen—free desserts, so she's buying whatever Gracie likes. NO SWEAT. My mom is going to pack me safe mini cupcakes that are peanut free and tree-nut free. ☺

Who's gonna hold my epinephrine? I can't jump with my epinephrine! They'll get in the way of my fun. ☹

My mom is coming! Gracie's mom even offered to hold my epinephrine in case my mom has to leave. My mom has shown me how to use it many times too. ☺ Epinephrine can save my life! It has medicine in it to help me breathe better and reduce any swelling if I accidentally eat a peanut or tree nut. Gracie's mom also said she'll make sure all the kids wash their hands before and after they eat. You just never know if anyone has eaten anything with nuts during the party!

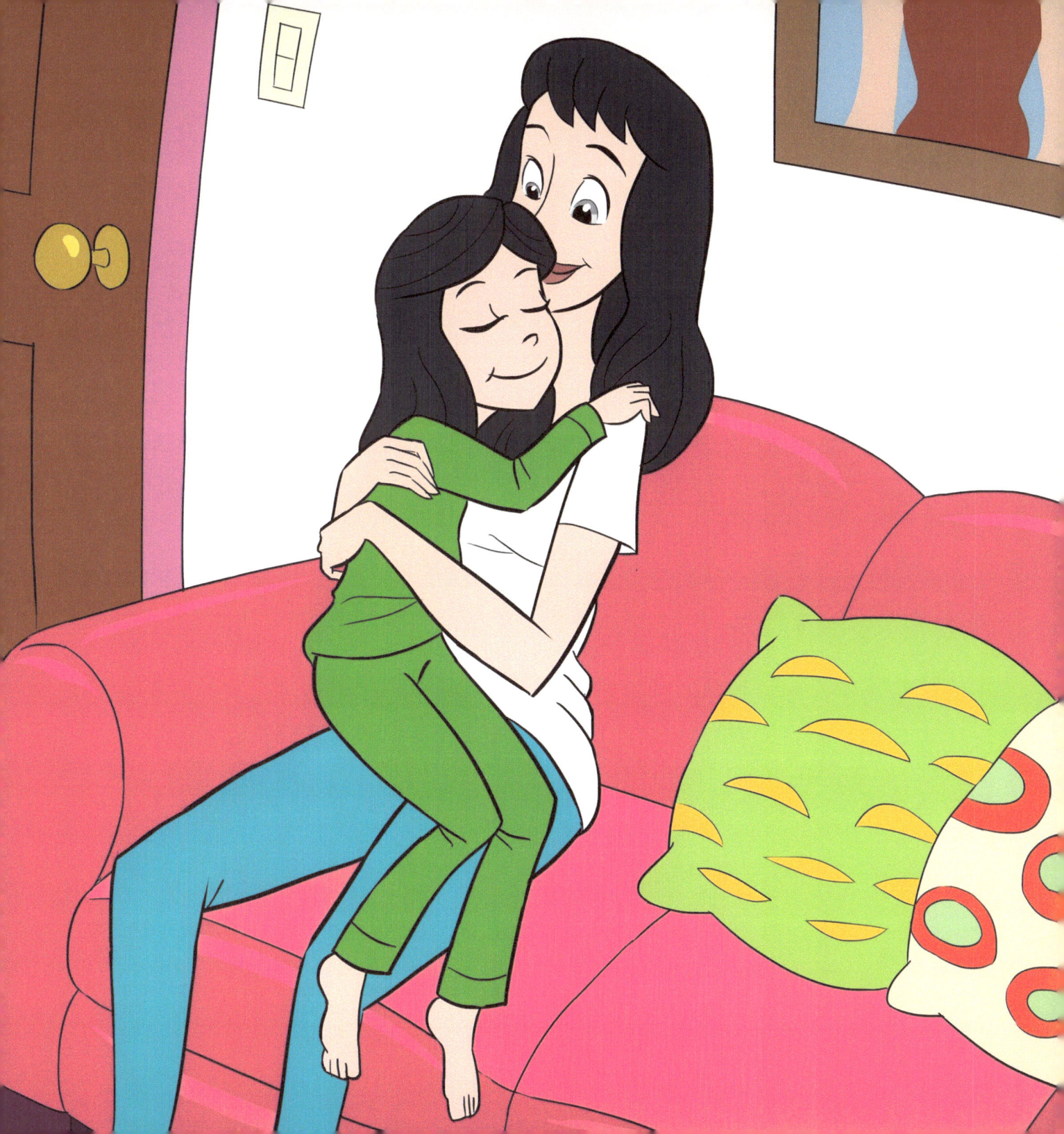

~WEDNESDAY~

Dear Diary,

I'm going to Sportsmania right after school on Friday to buy Gracie the cooolest gift ever. Wait till she sees the card I made for her!

So far, 11 girls are coming to the party. I can't wait!

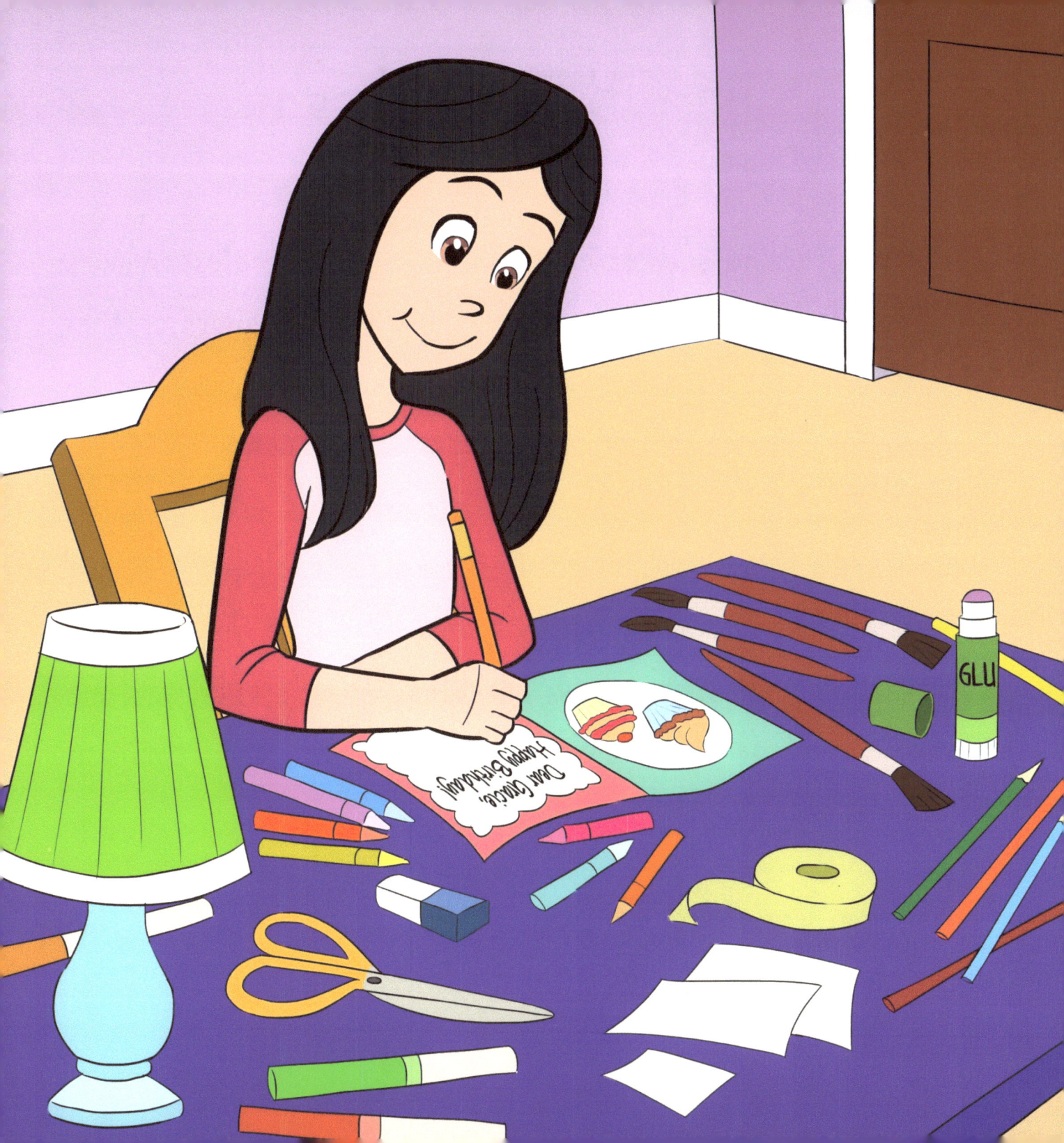

~ THURSDAY ~

Dear Diary,

I'm not feeling so worried about my food allergies anymore. My friends know I can't have anything with peanuts or tree nuts. Gosh, tree nuts are in so many foods. They're pistachios, almonds, pecans, hazelnuts, walnuts, and cashews! Whew! My friends hear all about keeping kids safe from food allergies at school, so they're used to it. They're so cool about it! They just want me to be safe. And it doesn't even bother them that I have food allergies. Gracie even told me that she reminded her mom about my allergies, and reminded her again and again. ☺

My mom was right! Friends will help keep me safe if they are truly my friends.

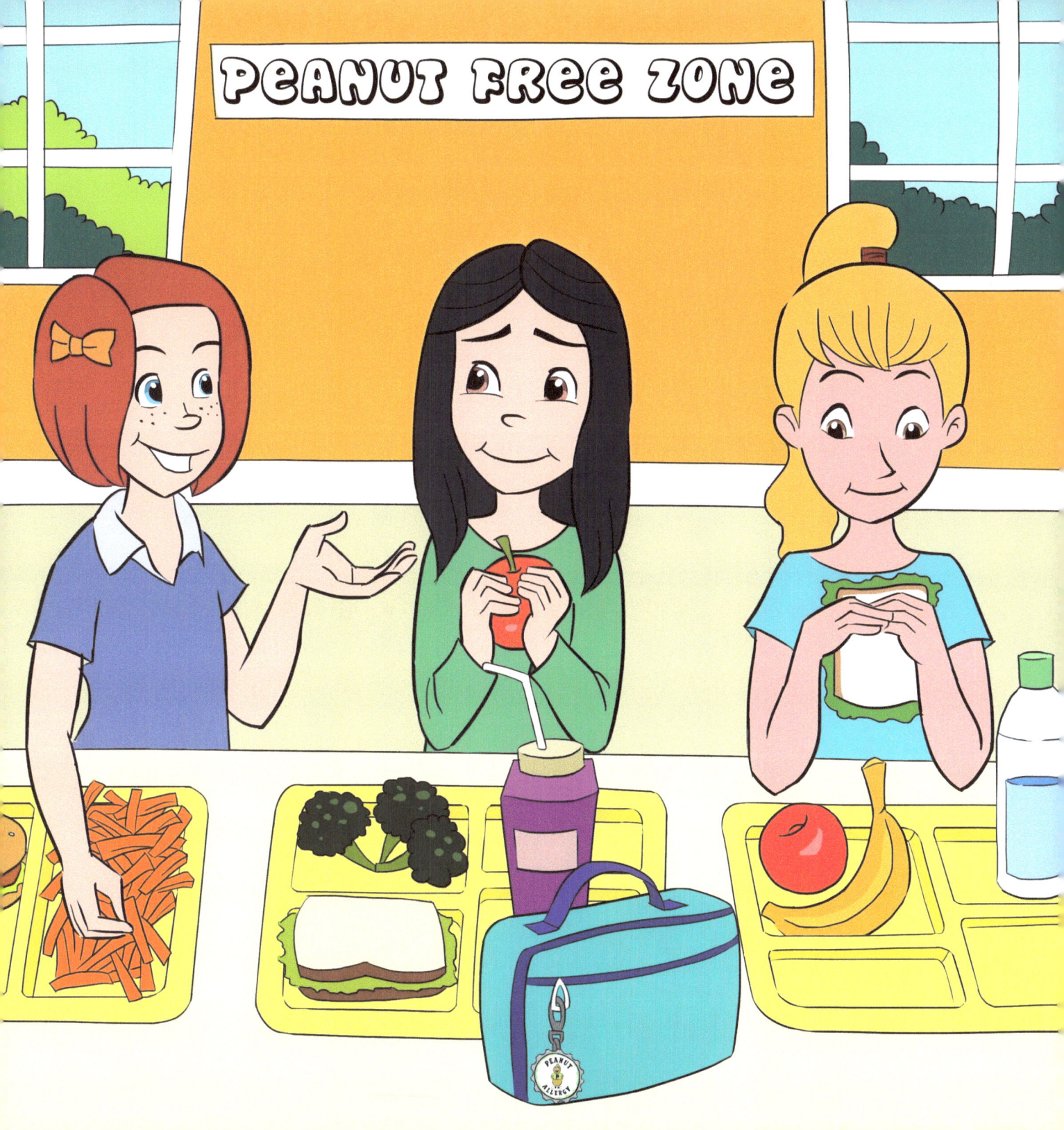

~FRIDAY~

Dear Diary,

I went to Sportsmania, Gracie's favorite store!

Gracie loves soccer, so I got the coolest blue soccer bag with a picture of a soccer ball in neon pink and green. I also filled the bag with the most delicious strawberry lip balms, crazy nail polish colors, and fancy headbands!

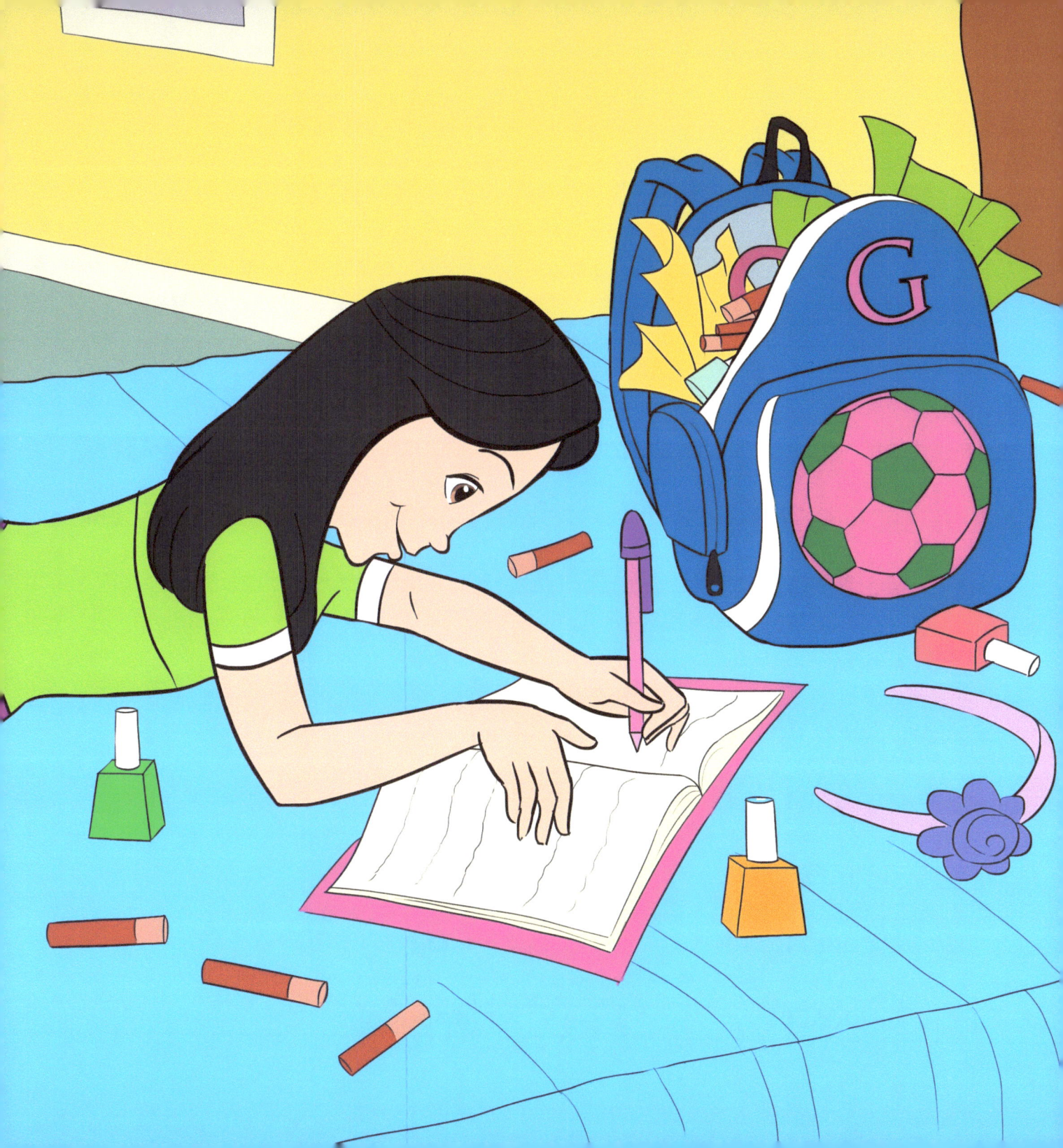

~ SATURDAY ~
IT'S PARTY TIME!

9:30 a.m.:

Counting down the hours until the party @ 12:30!

ANXIOUS EXCITED NERVOUS HAPPY

My mom made some delicious and mouth-watering chocolate and vanilla cupcakes with sprinkles on them. I can share them with my friends!

11:30 a.m.:

Gonna get dressed now. Woo-hoo!

Got my CHECKLIST

- ☑ Epinephrine
- ☑ Benadryl
- ☑ Cupcakes
- ☑ Gift
- ☑ Mama
- ☑ Happy girl

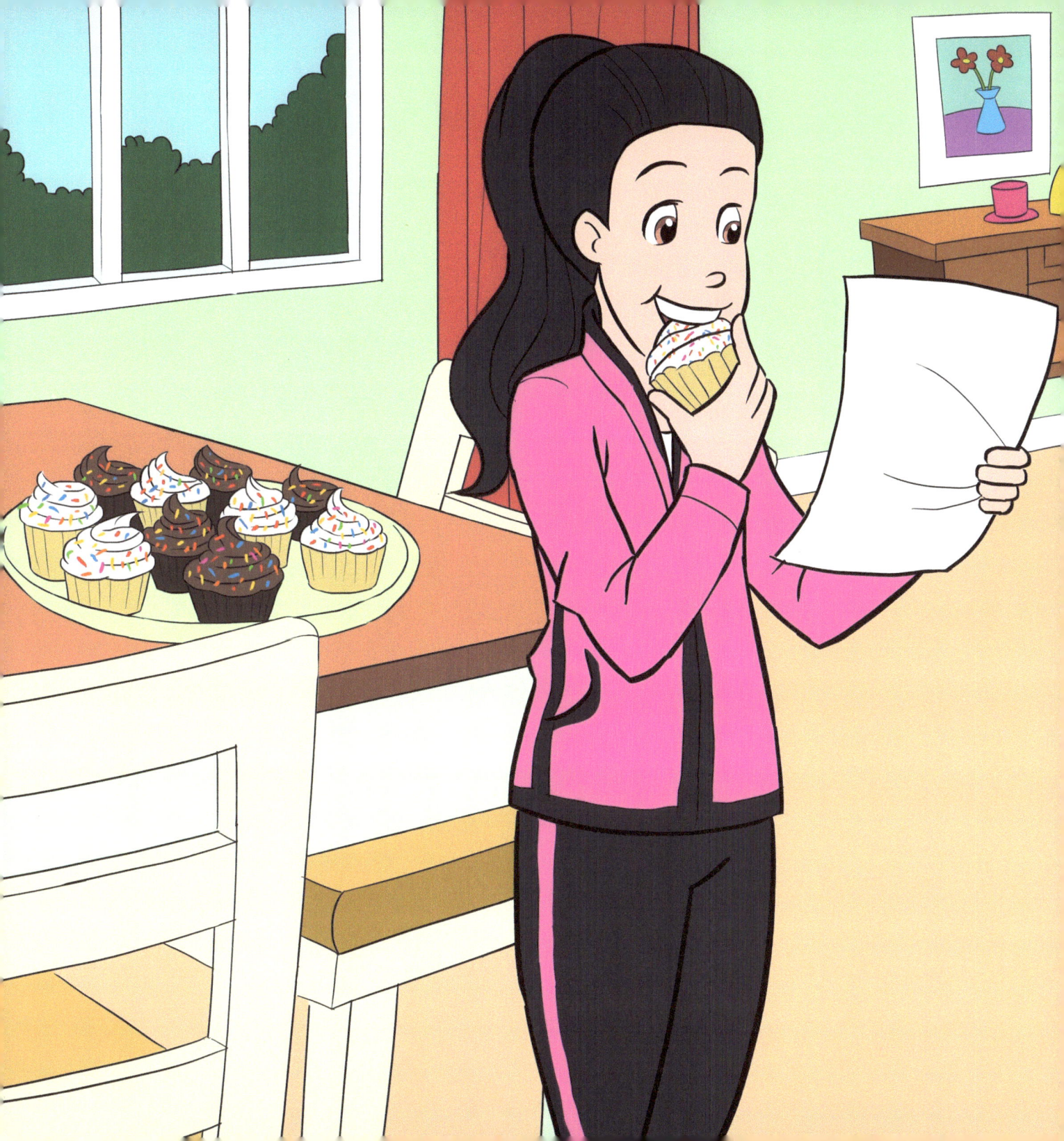

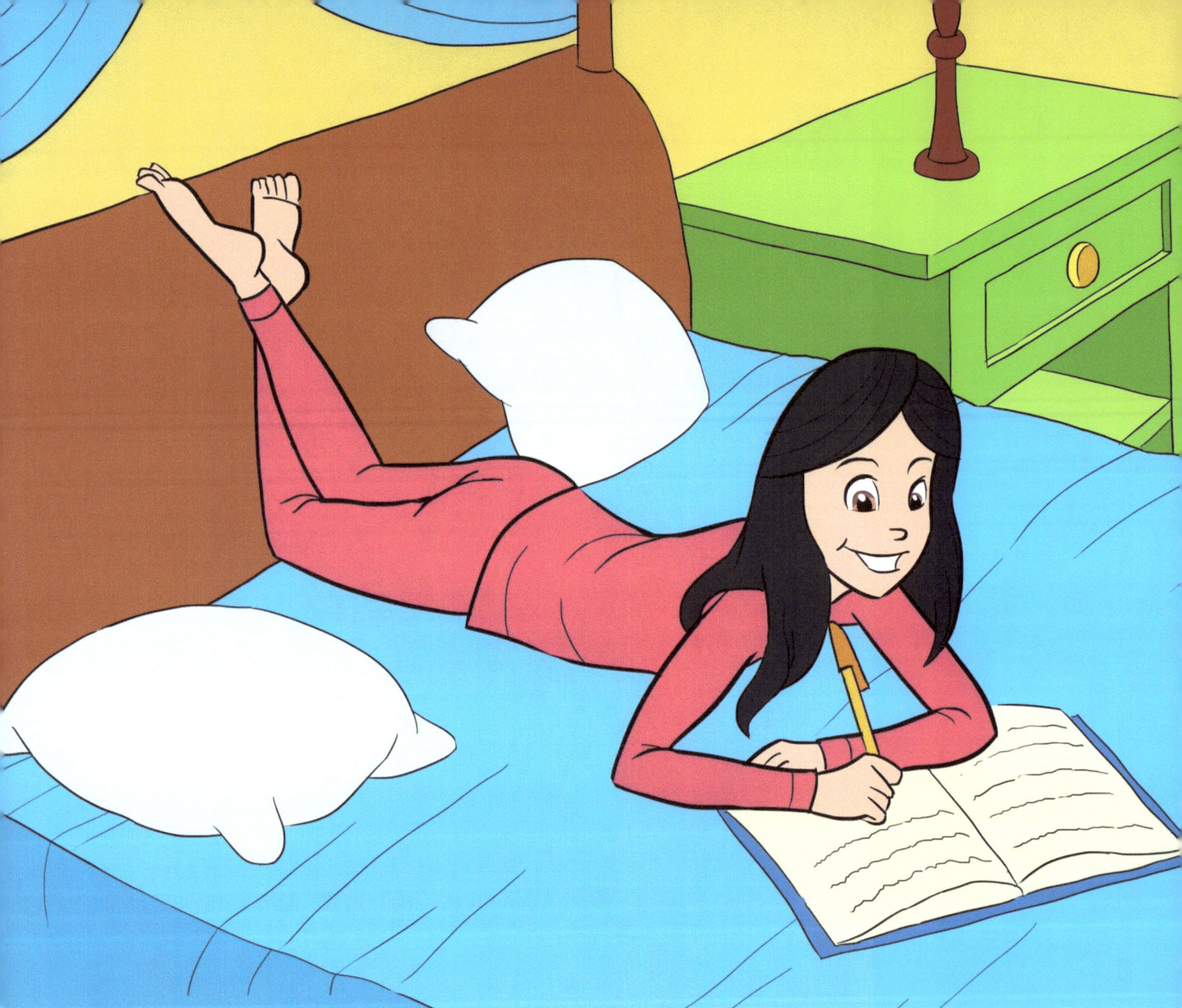

7p.m.:
I have never Jumped, Tumbled and Laughed so much in my life!
The party was spectacular!
I know it's important to keep me safe, but with family and friends by my side,

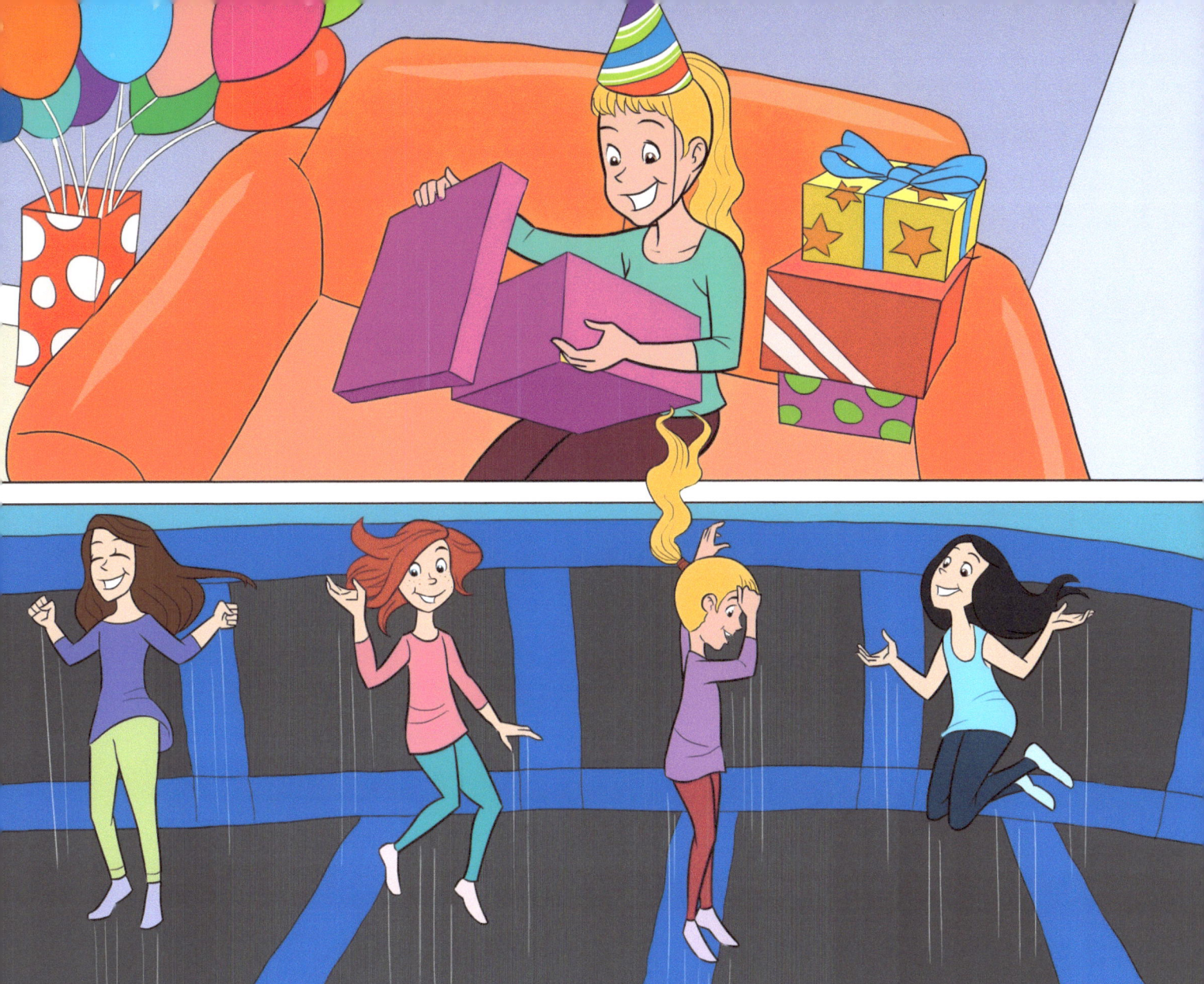

I'll never be afraid to go to another party again.
Oh wait! I think Tori is having a SLEEPOVER next month!
No sweat ~ I'll just come up with another plan! 😊

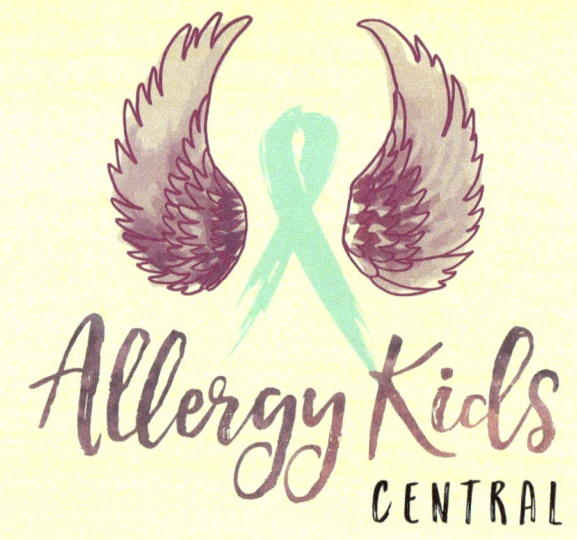

The End

To order one of our Alli-Caps, visit
www.AllergyKidsCentral.com.

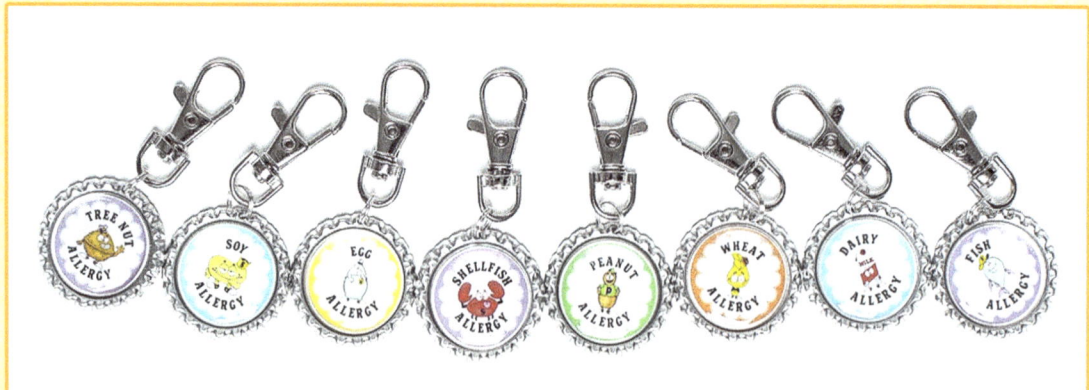

www.ingramcontent.com/pod-product-compliance
Lightning Source LLC
Chambersburg PA
CBHW060817290526
45792CB00005BB/1690